# DIET PLANNER

IT TAKES 21 DAYS TO MAKE
OR BREAK A HABIT

## THE FOUR STAGES OF HABIT

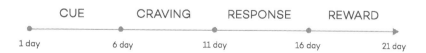

| CUE | CRAVING | RESPONSE | REWARD |

| 1 day | 6 day | 11 day | 16 day | 21 day |

# THREE MONTHS
# FROM NOW
# YOU WILL THANK
# YOURSELF

## MOTIVATIONAL AGREEMENT

MY GOALS

ACTIVITY/EXERCISE

CHANGING HABITS

YOUR SIGNATURE

# THE NEW YOU

KEEP YOUR BODY HYDRATED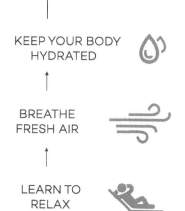

BREATHE FRESH AIR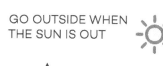

LEARN TO RELAX

GO OUTSIDE WHEN THE SUN IS OUT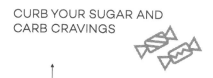

CURB YOUR SUGAR AND CARB CRAVINGS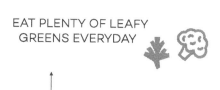

EAT PLENTY OF LEAFY GREENS EVERYDAY

LESS ANGER MORE LAUGHTER

FLOOD YOURSELF WITH EMPOWERING AFFIRMATIONS BEFORE STARTING YOUR DAY

GET TO BED ON TIME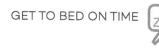

DO YOUR EXERCISE

STOP COMPARING YOURSELF TO OTHERS

DON'T BE TOO HARD ON YOURSELF

LESS WORDS MORE ACTION

MINIMIZE YOUR CONSUMPTION OF PROCESSED FOODS

TRANSITION FROM ACIDIC TO ALKALINE DIET

WATCH OUT FOR HIGH MERCURY FISHES

# HOW TO USE THIS PLANNER

DATE

MOTIVATIONAL
QUOTE

FOOD TIME
AND
DURATION

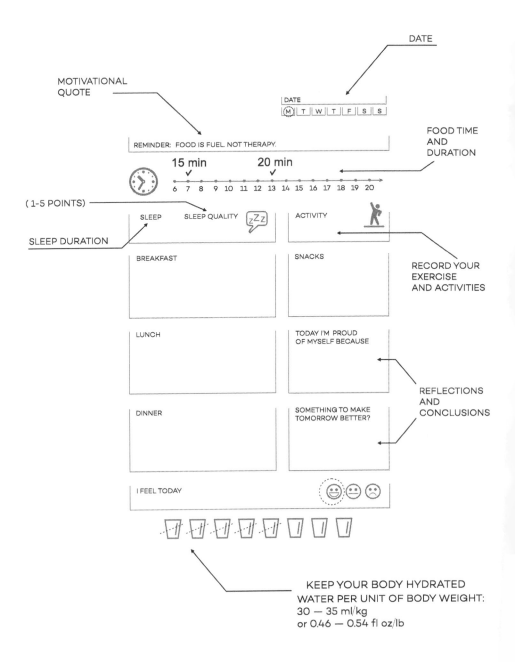

( 1-5 POINTS )

SLEEP DURATION

RECORD YOUR
EXERCISE
AND ACTIVITIES

REFLECTIONS
AND
CONCLUSIONS

KEEP YOUR BODY HYDRATED
WATER PER UNIT OF BODY WEIGHT:
30 — 35 ml/kg
or 0.46 — 0.54 fl oz/lb

# BODY PROGRESS

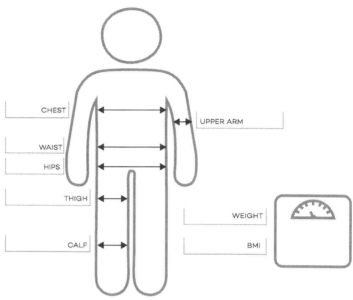

CHEST
UPPER ARM
WAIST
HIPS
THIGH
WEIGHT
CALF
BMI

# WEEK 1-4

| GOAL TRACKER | WEEK 1 | WEEK 2 | WEEK 3 | WEEK 4 |
|---|---|---|---|---|
| UPPER ARM | | | | |
| CHEST | | | | |
| WAIST | | | | |
| HIPS | | | | |
| THIGH | | | | |
| CALF | | | | |
| WEIGHT | | | | |

# WEEK 5-8

| GOAL TRACKER | WEEK 5 | WEEK 6 | WEEK 7 | WEEK 8 |
|---|---|---|---|---|
| UPPER ARM | | | | |
| CHEST | | | | |
| WAIST | | | | |
| HIPS | | | | |
| THIGH | | | | |
| CALF | | | | |
| WEIGHT | | | | |

2,2 mln ♥

# WEEK 9-12

| GOAL TRACKER | WEEK 9 | WEEK 10 | WEEK 11 | WEEK 12 |
|---|---|---|---|---|
| UPPER ARM | | | | |
| CHEST | | | | |
| WAIST | | | | |
| HIPS | | | | |
| THIGH | | | | |
| CALF | | | | |
| WEIGHT | | | | |

# WEEK 1 MEAL IDEAS

BREAKFAST

LUNCH

DINNER

SNACKS

**MONDAY**

BREAKFAST

LUNCH

DINNER

SNACKS

**TUESDAY**

BREAKFAST

LUNCH

DINNER

SNACKS

**WEDNESDAY**

BREAKFAST

LUNCH

DINNER

SNACKS

**THURSDAY**

BREAKFAST

LUNCH

DINNER

SNACKS

**FRIDAY**

BREAKFAST

LUNCH

DINNER

SNACKS

**SATURDAY**

BREAKFAST

LUNCH

DINNER

SNACKS

**SUNDAY**

SHOPPING LIST

# DAY 1

REMINDER: FOOD IS FUEL. NOT THERAPY.

 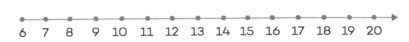

6  7  8  9  10  11  12  13  14  15  16  17  18  19  20

SLEEP    SLEEP QUALITY

ACTIVITY

BREAKFAST

SNACKS

LUNCH

TODAY I'M PROUD
OF MYSELF BECAUSE

DINNER

SOMETHING TO MAKE
TOMORROW BETTER?

I FEEL TODAY

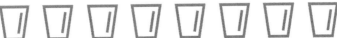

# DAY 2

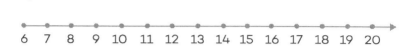

DATE

| M | T | W | T | F | S | S |

Get started as if you are motivated. Pretend. And the motivation will come!

6  7  8  9  10  11  12  13  14  15  16  17  18  19  20

SLEEP    SLEEP QUALITY

ACTIVITY

BREAKFAST

SNACKS

LUNCH

TODAY I'M PROUD
OF MYSELF BECAUSE

DINNER

SOMETHING TO MAKE
TOMORROW BETTER?

I FEEL TODAY

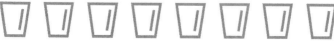

# DAY 3

The best project you'll ever work on is YOU.

 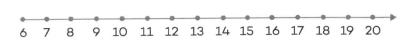

6  7  8  9  10  11  12  13  14  15  16  17  18  19  20

| SLEEP | SLEEP QUALITY  | ACTIVITY  |
|---|---|---|

BREAKFAST

SNACKS

LUNCH

TODAY I'M PROUD
OF MYSELF BECAUSE

DINNER

SOMETHING TO MAKE
TOMORROW BETTER?

I FEEL TODAY

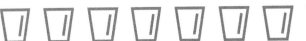

# DAY 4

Success is the sum of small efforts, repeated day-in and day-out.

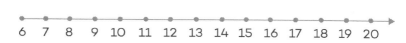

6 7 8 9 10 11 12 13 14 15 16 17 18 19 20

SLEEP      SLEEP QUALITY

ACTIVITY

BREAKFAST

SNACKS

LUNCH

TODAY I'M PROUD
OF MYSELF BECAUSE

DINNER

SOMETHING TO MAKE
TOMORROW BETTER?

I FEEL TODAY

# DAY 5

Only I can change my lfe, no one can do it for me.

 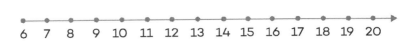

6  7  8  9  10  11  12  13  14  15  16  17  18  19  20

SLEEP        SLEEP QUALITY

ACTIVITY

BREAKFAST

SNACKS

LUNCH

TODAY I'M PROUD
OF MYSELF BECAUSE

DINNER

SOMETHING TO MAKE
TOMORROW BETTER?

I FEEL TODAY

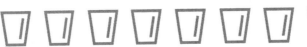

# DAY 6

Slow and steady wins the race.

 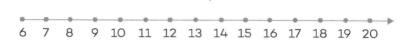

6   7   8   9   10   11   12   13   14   15   16   17   18   19   20

| SLEEP | SLEEP QUALITY  | ACTIVITY  |
|---|---|

BREAKFAST

SNACKS

LUNCH

TODAY I'M PROUD
OF MYSELF BECAUSE

DINNER

SOMETHING TO MAKE
TOMORROW BETTER?

I FEEL TODAY

# DAY 7

DATE

| M | T | W | T | F | S | S |
|---|---|---|---|---|---|---|

The struggle you are in today is developing the strength you need for tomorrow.

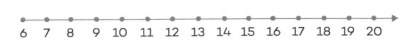

6  7  8  9  10  11  12  13  14  15  16  17  18  19  20

SLEEP     SLEEP QUALITY

ACTIVITY

BREAKFAST

SNACKS

LUNCH

TODAY I'M PROUD OF MYSELF BECAUSE

DINNER

SOMETHING TO MAKE TOMORROW BETTER?

I FEEL TODAY

# WEEK 2 MEAL IDEAS

BREAKFAST

LUNCH

DINNER

SNACKS

MONDAY

BREAKFAST

LUNCH

DINNER

SNACKS

TUESDAY

BREAKFAST

LUNCH

DINNER

SNACKS

WEDNESDAY

BREAKFAST

LUNCH

DINNER

SNACKS

THURSDAY

BREAKFAST

LUNCH

DINNER

SNACKS

FRIDAY

BREAKFAST

LUNCH

DINNER

SNACKS

SATURDAY

BREAKFAST

LUNCH

DINNER

SNACKS

SUNDAY

SHOPPING LIST

# DAY 8

Wow, I really regret that workout, said no one ever.

 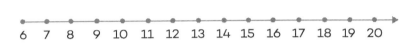

6  7  8  9  10  11  12  13  14  15  16  17  18  19  20

SLEEP        SLEEP QUALITY

ACTIVITY

BREAKFAST

SNACKS

LUNCH

TODAY I'M PROUD
OF MYSELF BECAUSE

DINNER

SOMETHING TO MAKE
TOMORROW BETTER?

I FEEL TODAY

# DAY 9

You are only limited to what you push yourself to, you know?
You can always get better.

 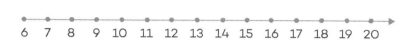

6  7  8  9  10  11  12  13  14  15  16  17  18  19  20

SLEEP          SLEEP QUALITY           ACTIVITY

BREAKFAST          SNACKS

LUNCH          TODAY I'M PROUD
OF MYSELF BECAUSE

DINNER          SOMETHING TO MAKE
TOMORROW BETTER?

I FEEL TODAY

# DAY 10

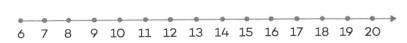

DATE
| M | T | W | T | F | S | S |
|---|---|---|---|---|---|---|

Your faith can move mountains and your doubt can create them.

 6  7  8  9  10  11  12  13  14  15  16  17  18  19  20

SLEEP    SLEEP QUALITY

ACTIVITY

BREAKFAST

SNACKS

LUNCH

TODAY I'M PROUD
OF MYSELF BECAUSE

DINNER

SOMETHING TO MAKE
TOMORROW BETTER?

I FEEL TODAY

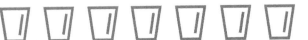

# DAY 11

When you want to give up, remember why you started.

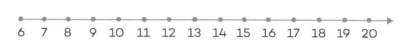

6  7  8  9  10  11  12  13  14  15  16  17  18  19  20

SLEEP    SLEEP QUALITY

ACTIVITY

BREAKFAST

SNACKS

LUNCH

TODAY I'M PROUD
OF MYSELF BECAUSE

DINNER

SOMETHING TO MAKE
TOMORROW BETTER?

I FEEL TODAY

# DAY 12

DATE

| M | T | W | T | F | S | S |
|---|---|---|---|---|---|---|

If you keep going you won't regret it. If you give up you will.

 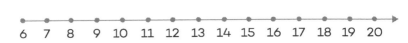

6  7  8  9  10  11  12  13  14  15  16  17  18  19  20

SLEEP    SLEEP QUALITY

ACTIVITY

BREAKFAST

SNACKS

LUNCH

TODAY I'M PROUD
OF MYSELF BECAUSE

DINNER

SOMETHING TO MAKE
TOMORROW BETTER?

I FEEL TODAY

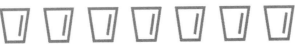

# DAY 13

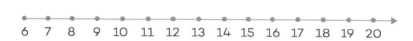

DATE

| M | T | W | T | F | S | S |
|---|---|---|---|---|---|---|

Take action!

  6  7  8  9  10  11  12  13  14  15  16  17  18  19  20

SLEEP    SLEEP QUALITY

ACTIVITY

BREAKFAST

SNACKS

LUNCH

TODAY I'M PROUD
OF MYSELF BECAUSE

DINNER

SOMETHING TO MAKE
TOMORROW BETTER?

I FEEL TODAY

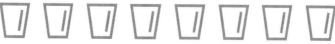

# DAY 14

The only bad workout is the one that didn't happen.

 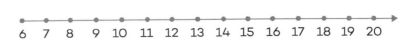

6 7 8 9 10 11 12 13 14 15 16 17 18 19 20

SLEEP    SLEEP QUALITY

ACTIVITY

BREAKFAST

SNACKS

LUNCH

TODAY I'M PROUD
OF MYSELF BECAUSE

DINNER

SOMETHING TO MAKE
TOMORROW BETTER?

I FEEL TODAY

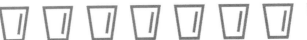

# WEEK 3 MEAL IDEAS

| | MONDAY |
|---|---|
| BREAKFAST | |
| LUNCH | |
| DINNER | |
| SNACKS | |

| | TUESDAY |
|---|---|
| BREAKFAST | |
| LUNCH | |
| DINNER | |
| SNACKS | |

| | WEDNESDAY |
|---|---|
| BREAKFAST | |
| LUNCH | |
| DINNER | |
| SNACKS | |

| | THURSDAY |
|---|---|
| BREAKFAST | |
| LUNCH | |
| DINNER | |
| SNACKS | |

| | FRIDAY |
|---|---|
| BREAKFAST | |
| LUNCH | |
| DINNER | |
| SNACKS | |

| | SATURDAY |
|---|---|
| BREAKFAST | |
| LUNCH | |
| DINNER | |
| SNACKS | |

| | SUNDAY |
|---|---|
| BREAKFAST | |
| LUNCH | |
| DINNER | |
| SNACKS | |

SHOPPING LIST

# DAY 15

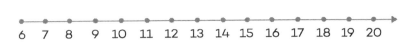

DATE

| M | T | W | T | F | S | S |
|---|---|---|---|---|---|---|

Being challenged in life is inevitable. Being defeated is optional.

6  7  8  9  10  11  12  13  14  15  16  17  18  19  20

SLEEP            SLEEP QUALITY            ACTIVITY

BREAKFAST            SNACKS

LUNCH            TODAY I'M PROUD
OF MYSELF BECAUSE

DINNER            SOMETHING TO MAKE
TOMORROW BETTER?

I FEEL TODAY

# DAY 16

Think of that feeling you'll get when you've reached your goal weight.

  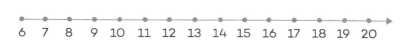

6  7  8  9  10  11  12  13  14  15  16  17  18  19  20

SLEEP    SLEEP QUALITY

ACTIVITY

BREAKFAST

SNACKS

LUNCH

TODAY I'M PROUD
OF MYSELF BECAUSE

DINNER

SOMETHING TO MAKE
TOMORROW BETTER?

I FEEL TODAY

# DAY 17

And Yes, it is possible, and No, it isn't easy.

 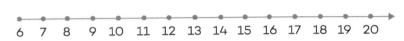

6  7  8  9  10  11  12  13  14  15  16  17  18  19  20

SLEEP    SLEEP QUALITY

ACTIVITY

BREAKFAST

SNACKS

LUNCH

TODAY I'M PROUD
OF MYSELF BECAUSE

DINNER

SOMETHING TO MAKE
TOMORROW BETTER?

I FEEL TODAY

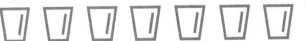

# DAY 18

DATE
M T W T F S S

It's not about having time. It's about making time.

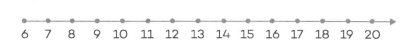

6 7 8 9 10 11 12 13 14 15 16 17 18 19 20

SLEEP   SLEEP QUALITY

ACTIVITY

BREAKFAST

SNACKS

LUNCH

TODAY I'M PROUD
OF MYSELF BECAUSE

DINNER

SOMETHING TO MAKE
TOMORROW BETTER?

I FEEL TODAY

# DAY 19

DATE
| M | T | W | T | F | S | S |

Be stronger than your excuses.

 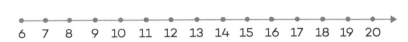

6  7  8  9  10  11  12  13  14  15  16  17  18  19  20

SLEEP    SLEEP QUALITY

ACTIVITY

BREAKFAST

SNACKS

LUNCH

TODAY I'M PROUD
OF MYSELF BECAUSE

DINNER

SOMETHING TO MAKE
TOMORROW BETTER?

I FEEL TODAY

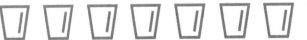

# DAY 20

DATE

| M | T | W | T | F | S | S |
|---|---|---|---|---|---|---|

Don't compare yourself to others.
Compare yourself to the person from yesterday.

6  7  8  9  10  11  12  13  14  15  16  17  18  19  20

SLEEP       SLEEP QUALITY

ACTIVITY

BREAKFAST

SNACKS

LUNCH

TODAY I'M PROUD
OF MYSELF BECAUSE

DINNER

SOMETHING TO MAKE
TOMORROW BETTER?

I FEEL TODAY

# DAY 21

DATE
| M | T | W | T | F | S | S |
|---|---|---|---|---|---|---|
|   |   |   |   |   |   |   |

A huge part of losing weight is believing you can do it
and realizing it's not going to happen overnight.

 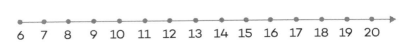

6  7  8  9  10  11  12  13  14  15  16  17  18  19  20

SLEEP        SLEEP QUALITY          ACTIVITY

BREAKFAST

SNACKS

LUNCH

TODAY I'M PROUD
OF MYSELF BECAUSE

DINNER

SOMETHING TO MAKE
TOMORROW BETTER?

I FEEL TODAY

# WEEK 4 MEAL IDEAS

BREAKFAST

LUNCH

DINNER

SNACKS

MONDAY

BREAKFAST

LUNCH

DINNER

SNACKS

TUESDAY

BREAKFAST

LUNCH

DINNER

SNACKS

WEDNESDAY

BREAKFAST

LUNCH

DINNER

SNACKS

THURSDAY

BREAKFAST

LUNCH

DINNER

SNACKS

FRIDAY

BREAKFAST

LUNCH

DINNER

SNACKS

SATURDAY

BREAKFAST

LUNCH

DINNER

SNACKS

SUNDAY

SHOPPING LIST

# DAY 22

Look in the mirror, that's your competition.

 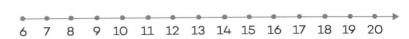

6  7  8  9  10  11  12  13  14  15  16  17  18  19  20

| SLEEP | SLEEP QUALITY  | ACTIVITY  |

BREAKFAST

SNACKS

LUNCH

TODAY I'M PROUD OF MYSELF BECAUSE

DINNER

SOMETHING TO MAKE TOMORROW BETTER?

I FEEL TODAY

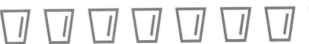

# DAY 23

You don't have to be great to start, but you have to start to be great.

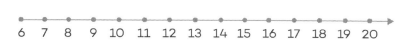

6  7  8  9  10  11  12  13  14  15  16  17  18  19  20

SLEEP          SLEEP QUALITY

ACTIVITY

BREAKFAST

SNACKS

LUNCH

TODAY I'M PROUD
OF MYSELF BECAUSE

DINNER

SOMETHING TO MAKE
TOMORROW BETTER?

I FEEL TODAY

# DAY 24

Weight loss is not meant to be a sprint. It's a marathon.

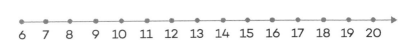
6  7  8  9  10  11  12  13  14  15  16  17  18  19  20

SLEEP          SLEEP QUALITY

ACTIVITY

BREAKFAST

SNACKS

LUNCH

TODAY I'M PROUD
OF MYSELF BECAUSE

DINNER

SOMETHING TO MAKE
TOMORROW BETTER?

I FEEL TODAY

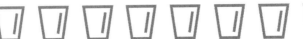

# DAY 25

DATE

| M | T | W | T | F | S | S |
|---|---|---|---|---|---|---|

Yesterday you said tomorrow.

 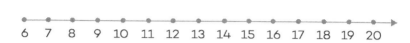

6  7  8  9  10  11  12  13  14  15  16  17  18  19  20

SLEEP        SLEEP QUALITY

ACTIVITY

BREAKFAST

SNACKS

LUNCH

TODAY I'M PROUD
OF MYSELF BECAUSE

DINNER

SOMETHING TO MAKE
TOMORROW BETTER?

I FEEL TODAY

# DAY 26

DATE

| M | T | W | T | F | S | S |
|---|---|---|---|---|---|---|

Your only limit is YOU.

 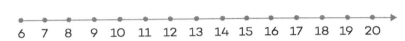

6  7  8  9  10  11  12  13  14  15  16  17  18  19  20

SLEEP     SLEEP QUALITY

ACTIVITY

BREAKFAST

SNACKS

LUNCH

TODAY I'M PROUD
OF MYSELF BECAUSE

DINNER

SOMETHING TO MAKE
TOMORROW BETTER?

I FEEL TODAY

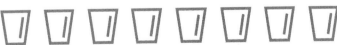

# DAY 27

DATE
M | T | W | T | F | S | S

You are stronger than you know.

 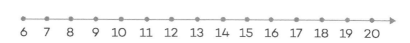

6  7  8  9  10  11  12  13  14  15  16  17  18  19  20

SLEEP     SLEEP QUALITY

ACTIVITY

BREAKFAST

SNACKS

LUNCH

TODAY I'M PROUD
OF MYSELF BECAUSE

DINNER

SOMETHING TO MAKE
TOMORROW BETTER?

I FEEL TODAY

# DAY 28

Dear stomach. You're bored. Not hungry. So shut up!

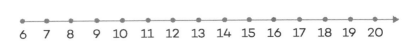

6  7  8  9  10  11  12  13  14  15  16  17  18  19  20

SLEEP    SLEEP QUALITY

ACTIVITY

BREAKFAST

SNACKS

LUNCH

TODAY I'M PROUD
OF MYSELF BECAUSE

DINNER

SOMETHING TO MAKE
TOMORROW BETTER?

I FEEL TODAY

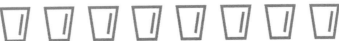

# WEEK 5 MEAL IDEAS

| | | |
|---|---|---|
| BREAKFAST | | |
| LUNCH | | |
| DINNER | MONDAY | SHOPPING LIST |
| SNACKS | | |
| BREAKFAST | | |
| LUNCH | | |
| DINNER | TUESDAY | |
| SNACKS | | |
| BREAKFAST | | |
| LUNCH | | |
| DINNER | WEDNESDAY | |
| SNACKS | | |
| BREAKFAST | | |
| LUNCH | | |
| DINNER | THURSDAY | |
| SNACKS | | |
| BREAKFAST | | |
| LUNCH | | |
| DINNER | FRIDAY | |
| SNACKS | | |
| BREAKFAST | | |
| LUNCH | | |
| DINNER | SATURDAY | |
| SNACKS | | |
| BREAKFAST | | |
| LUNCH | | |
| DINNER | SUNDAY | |
| SNACKS | | |

# DAY 29

The groundwork of all happiness is health.

 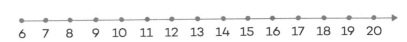

6  7  8  9  10  11  12  13  14  15  16  17  18  19  20

SLEEP     SLEEP QUALITY

ACTIVITY

BREAKFAST

SNACKS

LUNCH

TODAY I'M PROUD
OF MYSELF BECAUSE

DINNER

SOMETHING TO MAKE
TOMORROW BETTER?

I FEEL TODAY

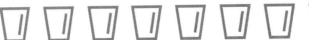

# DAY 30

DATE

| M | T | W | T | F | S | S |
|---|---|---|---|---|---|---|

Small steps baby, small steps.

 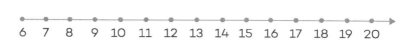

6  7  8  9  10  11  12  13  14  15  16  17  18  19  20

| SLEEP | SLEEP QUALITY  | ACTIVITY  |
|---|---|---|

| BREAKFAST | SNACKS |
|---|---|

| LUNCH | TODAY I'M PROUD OF MYSELF BECAUSE |
|---|---|

| DINNER | SOMETHING TO MAKE TOMORROW BETTER? |
|---|---|

I FEEL TODAY

# DAY 31

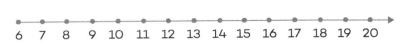

DATE

| M | T | W | T | F | S | S |
|---|---|---|---|---|---|---|

It took more than a day to put it on. It will take more than a day to take it off.

6  7  8  9  10  11  12  13  14  15  16  17  18  19  20

SLEEP        SLEEP QUALITY

ACTIVITY

BREAKFAST

SNACKS

LUNCH

TODAY I'M PROUD OF MYSELF BECAUSE

DINNER

SOMETHING TO MAKE TOMORROW BETTER?

I FEEL TODAY

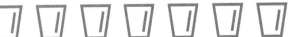

# DAY 32

If you keep good food in your fridge, you will eat good food.

 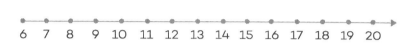

6  7  8  9  10  11  12  13  14  15  16  17  18  19  20

SLEEP        SLEEP QUALITY

ACTIVITY

BREAKFAST

SNACKS

LUNCH

TODAY I'M PROUD
OF MYSELF BECAUSE

DINNER

SOMETHING TO MAKE
TOMORROW BETTER?

I FEEL TODAY

# DAY 33

DATE

| M | T | W | T | F | S | S |
|---|---|---|---|---|---|---|
|   |   |   |   |   |   |   |

It takes five minutes to consume 500 calories.
It takes two hours to burn them off.

6  7  8  9  10  11  12  13  14  15  16  17  18  19  20

SLEEP     SLEEP QUALITY

ACTIVITY

BREAKFAST

SNACKS

LUNCH

TODAY I'M PROUD
OF MYSELF BECAUSE

DINNER

SOMETHING TO MAKE
TOMORROW BETTER?

I FEEL TODAY

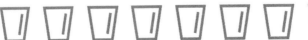

# DAY 34

One must eat to live, not live to eat.

 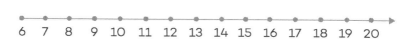

6 7 8 9 10 11 12 13 14 15 16 17 18 19 20

SLEEP    SLEEP QUALITY

ACTIVITY

BREAKFAST

SNACKS

LUNCH

TODAY I'M PROUD
OF MYSELF BECAUSE

DINNER

SOMETHING TO MAKE
TOMORROW BETTER?

I FEEL TODAY

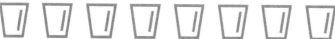

# DAY 35

Exercising should be about rewarding the body with endorphins and strength. Not about punishing your body for what you've eaten.

 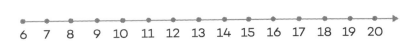

SLEEP    SLEEP QUALITY

ACTIVITY

BREAKFAST

SNACKS

LUNCH

TODAY I'M PROUD OF MYSELF BECAUSE

DINNER

SOMETHING TO MAKE TOMORROW BETTER?

I FEEL TODAY

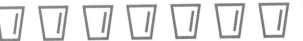

# WEEK 6 MEAL IDEAS

| | |
|---|---|
| BREAKFAST<br>LUNCH<br>DINNER<br>SNACKS | MONDAY |
| BREAKFAST<br>LUNCH<br>DINNER<br>SNACKS | TUESDAY |
| BREAKFAST<br>LUNCH<br>DINNER<br>SNACKS | WEDNESDAY |
| BREAKFAST<br>LUNCH<br>DINNER<br>SNACKS | THURSDAY |
| BREAKFAST<br>LUNCH<br>DINNER<br>SNACKS | FRIDAY |
| BREAKFAST<br>LUNCH<br>DINNER<br>SNACKS | SATURDAY |
| BREAKFAST<br>LUNCH<br>DINNER<br>SNACKS | SUNDAY |

SHOPPING LIST

# DAY 36

DATE

| M | T | W | T | F | S | S |
|---|---|---|---|---|---|---|
|   |   |   |   |   |   |   |

Don't dig your grave with your own knife and fork.

  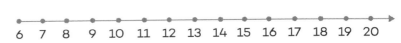

6  7  8  9  10  11  12  13  14  15  16  17  18  19  20

SLEEP          SLEEP QUALITY

ACTIVITY

BREAKFAST

SNACKS

LUNCH

TODAY I'M PROUD
OF MYSELF BECAUSE

DINNER

SOMETHING TO MAKE
TOMORROW BETTER?

I FEEL TODAY

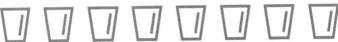

# DAY 37

Never lose your sense of wonder.

 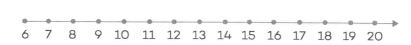

6  7  8  9  10  11  12  13  14  15  16  17  18  19  20

SLEEP          SLEEP QUALITY                    ACTIVITY

BREAKFAST          SNACKS

LUNCH          TODAY I'M PROUD OF MYSELF BECAUSE

DINNER          SOMETHING TO MAKE TOMORROW BETTER?

I FEEL TODAY

 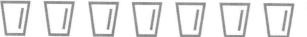

# DAY 38

Imperfection is not a flaw.

 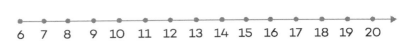

6  7  8  9  10  11  12  13  14  15  16  17  18  19  20

SLEEP        SLEEP QUALITY

ACTIVITY

BREAKFAST

SNACKS

LUNCH

TODAY I'M PROUD
OF MYSELF BECAUSE

DINNER

SOMETHING TO MAKE
TOMORROW BETTER?

I FEEL TODAY

      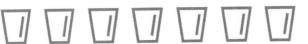

# DAY 39

DATE

| M | T | W | T | F | S | S |
|---|---|---|---|---|---|---|
|   |   |   |   |   |   |   |

Your goals, minus your doubts, equal your reality.

 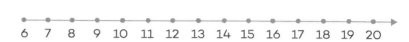

6  7  8  9  10  11  12  13  14  15  16  17  18  19  20

SLEEP      SLEEP QUALITY

ACTIVITY

BREAKFAST

SNACKS

LUNCH

TODAY I'M PROUD
OF MYSELF BECAUSE

DINNER

SOMETHING TO MAKE
TOMORROW BETTER?

I FEEL TODAY

# DAY 40

| M | T | W | T | F | S | S |
|---|---|---|---|---|---|---|

An optimist is a person who starts a new diet on Thanksgiving Day.

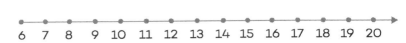
6  7  8  9  10  11  12  13  14  15  16  17  18  19  20

SLEEP    SLEEP QUALITY

ACTIVITY

BREAKFAST

SNACKS

LUNCH

TODAY I'M PROUD
OF MYSELF BECAUSE

DINNER

SOMETHING TO MAKE
TOMORROW BETTER?

I FEEL TODAY

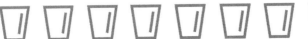

# DAY 41

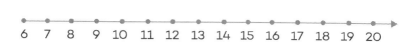

DATE

| M | T | W | T | F | S | S |
|---|---|---|---|---|---|---|

You don't drown by falling in water. You drown by staying there.

 6 7 8 9 10 11 12 13 14 15 16 17 18 19 20

SLEEP      SLEEP QUALITY

ACTIVITY

BREAKFAST

SNACKS

LUNCH

TODAY I'M PROUD
OF MYSELF BECAUSE

DINNER

SOMETHING TO MAKE
TOMORROW BETTER?

I FEEL TODAY

# DAY 42

People have got to learn: if they don't have cookies in the cookie jar, they can't eat cookies.

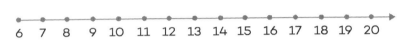

6  7  8  9  10  11  12  13  14  15  16  17  18  19  20

SLEEP    SLEEP QUALITY

ACTIVITY

BREAKFAST

SNACKS

LUNCH

TODAY I'M PROUD
OF MYSELF BECAUSE

DINNER

SOMETHING TO MAKE
TOMORROW BETTER?

I FEEL TODAY

 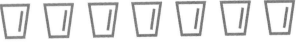

# WEEK 7 MEAL IDEAS

BREAKFAST

LUNCH

DINNER

SNACKS

MONDAY

BREAKFAST

LUNCH

DINNER

SNACKS

TUESDAY

BREAKFAST

LUNCH

DINNER

SNACKS

WEDNESDAY

BREAKFAST

LUNCH

DINNER

SNACKS

THURSDAY

BREAKFAST

LUNCH

DINNER

SNACKS

FRIDAY

BREAKFAST

LUNCH

DINNER

SNACKS

SATURDAY

BREAKFAST

LUNCH

DINNER

SNACKS

SUNDAY

SHOPPING LIST

# DAY 43

If it was about knowledge, we would all be skinny and rich.
It's not about what you know but what you do!

 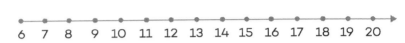

6  7  8  9  10  11  12  13  14  15  16  17  18  19  20

SLEEP          SLEEP QUALITY              ACTIVITY

BREAKFAST

SNACKS

LUNCH

TODAY I'M PROUD
OF MYSELF BECAUSE

DINNER

SOMETHING TO MAKE
TOMORROW BETTER?

I FEEL TODAY

      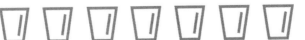

# DAY 44

DATE

| M | T | W | T | F | S | S |
|---|---|---|---|---|---|---|

Someone busier than you is running right now.

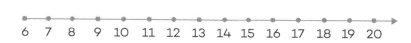

6  7  8  9  10  11  12  13  14  15  16  17  18  19  20

| SLEEP | SLEEP QUALITY  | ACTIVITY  |
|---|---|---|

BREAKFAST

SNACKS

LUNCH

TODAY I'M PROUD
OF MYSELF BECAUSE

DINNER

SOMETHING TO MAKE
TOMORROW BETTER?

I FEEL TODAY

# DAY 45

DATE
| M | T | W | T | F | S | S |
|---|---|---|---|---|---|---|

Working out is never convenient. But neither is illness, diabetes and obesity!

 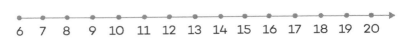

6 7 8 9 10 11 12 13 14 15 16 17 18 19 20

SLEEP        SLEEP QUALITY

ACTIVITY

BREAKFAST

SNACKS

LUNCH

TODAY I'M PROUD
OF MYSELF BECAUSE

DINNER

SOMETHING TO MAKE
TOMORROW BETTER?

I FEEL TODAY

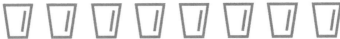

# DAY 46

DATE

| M | T | W | T | F | S | S |
|---|---|---|---|---|---|---|

I don't stop when I'm tired, I stop when I'M DONE!

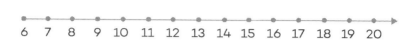

6  7  8  9  10  11  12  13  14  15  16  17  18  19  20

SLEEP          SLEEP QUALITY

ACTIVITY

BREAKFAST

SNACKS

LUNCH

TODAY I'M PROUD
OF MYSELF BECAUSE

DINNER

SOMETHING TO MAKE
TOMORROW BETTER?

I FEEL TODAY

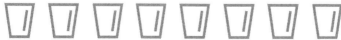

# DAY 47

I don't work hard because I hate my body. I workout because I love it!

 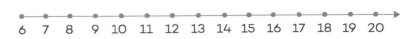

6  7  8  9  10  11  12  13  14  15  16  17  18  19  20

SLEEP        SLEEP QUALITY

ACTIVITY

BREAKFAST

SNACKS

LUNCH

TODAY I'M PROUD
OF MYSELF BECAUSE

DINNER

SOMETHING TO MAKE
TOMORROW BETTER?

I FEEL TODAY

# DAY 48

Get comfortable with being uncomfortable!

 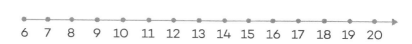

6  7  8  9  10  11  12  13  14  15  16  17  18  19  20

SLEEP          SLEEP QUALITY

ACTIVITY

BREAKFAST

SNACKS

LUNCH

TODAY I'M PROUD
OF MYSELF BECAUSE

DINNER

SOMETHING TO MAKE
TOMORROW BETTER?

I FEEL TODAY

# DAY 49

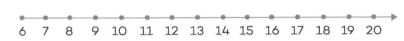

DATE

| M | T | W | T | F | S | S |
|---|---|---|---|---|---|---|

When it burns, is when you're just getting started.
That's when you get stronger!

 6 7 8 9 10 11 12 13 14 15 16 17 18 19 20

SLEEP    SLEEP QUALITY

ACTIVITY

BREAKFAST

SNACKS

LUNCH

TODAY I'M PROUD
OF MYSELF BECAUSE

DINNER

SOMETHING TO MAKE
TOMORROW BETTER?

I FEEL TODAY

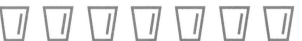

# WEEK 8 MEAL IDEAS

BREAKFAST

LUNCH

DINNER

SNACKS

**MONDAY**

BREAKFAST

LUNCH

DINNER

SNACKS

**TUESDAY**

BREAKFAST

LUNCH

DINNER

SNACKS

**WEDNESDAY**

BREAKFAST

LUNCH

DINNER

SNACKS

**THURSDAY**

BREAKFAST

LUNCH

DINNER

SNACKS

**FRIDAY**

BREAKFAST

LUNCH

DINNER

SNACKS

**SATURDAY**

BREAKFAST

LUNCH

DINNER

SNACKS

**SUNDAY**

SHOPPING LIST

# DAY 50

DATE
| M | T | W | T | F | S | S |
|---|---|---|---|---|---|---|

If you have 30 minutes for Facebook, you have 1 hour for the gym!

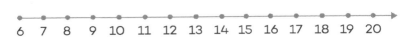

6  7  8  9  10  11  12  13  14  15  16  17  18  19  20

SLEEP        SLEEP QUALITY            ACTIVITY

BREAKFAST                                SNACKS

LUNCH                                    TODAY I'M PROUD
                                         OF MYSELF BECAUSE

DINNER                                   SOMETHING TO MAKE
                                         TOMORROW BETTER?

I FEEL TODAY

# DAY 51

DATE

| M | T | W | T | F | S | S |
|---|---|---|---|---|---|---|

The best way to predict your health is to create it.

 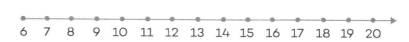

6  7  8  9  10  11  12  13  14  15  16  17  18  19  20

| SLEEP    SLEEP QUALITY  | ACTIVITY  |
|---|---|
| BREAKFAST | SNACKS |
| LUNCH | TODAY I'M PROUD OF MYSELF BECAUSE |
| DINNER | SOMETHING TO MAKE TOMORROW BETTER? |

I FEEL TODAY

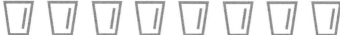

# DAY 52

You can't run from all your problems, but it will help you lose weight.

 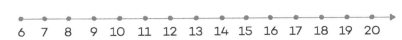

6 7 8 9 10 11 12 13 14 15 16 17 18 19 20

SLEEP        SLEEP QUALITY

ACTIVITY

BREAKFAST

SNACKS

LUNCH

TODAY I'M PROUD
OF MYSELF BECAUSE

DINNER

SOMETHING TO MAKE
TOMORROW BETTER?

I FEEL TODAY

 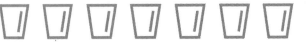

# DAY 53

M  T  W  T  F  S  S

Excuses don't burn calories.

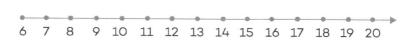

6  7  8  9  10  11  12  13  14  15  16  17  18  19  20

SLEEP        SLEEP QUALITY

ACTIVITY

BREAKFAST

SNACKS

LUNCH

TODAY I'M PROUD
OF MYSELF BECAUSE

DINNER

SOMETHING TO MAKE
TOMORROW BETTER?

I FEEL TODAY

# DAY 54

Your body hears everything your mind says. Keep going. You can!

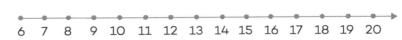

6  7  8  9  10  11  12  13  14  15  16  17  18  19  20

SLEEP          SLEEP QUALITY

ACTIVITY

BREAKFAST

SNACKS

LUNCH

TODAY I'M PROUD
OF MYSELF BECAUSE

DINNER

SOMETHING TO MAKE
TOMORROW BETTER?

I FEEL TODAY

 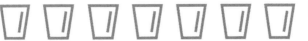

# DAY 55

Don't stop until you're proud.

 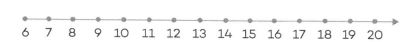

6  7  8  9  10  11  12  13  14  15  16  17  18  19  20

SLEEP          SLEEP QUALITY           ACTIVITY

BREAKFAST          SNACKS

LUNCH          TODAY I'M PROUD
OF MYSELF BECAUSE

DINNER          SOMETHING TO MAKE
TOMORROW BETTER?

I FEEL TODAY

# DAY 56

DATE

| M | T | W | T | F | S | S |

You don't have to go fast, you just have to go.

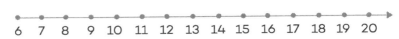

6   7   8   9   10   11   12   13   14   15   16   17   18   19   20

SLEEP        SLEEP QUALITY

ACTIVITY

BREAKFAST

SNACKS

LUNCH

TODAY I'M PROUD
OF MYSELF BECAUSE

DINNER

SOMETHING TO MAKE
TOMORROW BETTER?

I FEEL TODAY

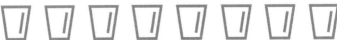

# WEEK 9 MEAL IDEAS

BREAKFAST

LUNCH

DINNER

SNACKS

MONDAY

BREAKFAST

LUNCH

DINNER

SNACKS

TUESDAY

BREAKFAST

LUNCH

DINNER

SNACKS

WEDNESDAY

BREAKFAST

LUNCH

DINNER

SNACKS

THURSDAY

BREAKFAST

LUNCH

DINNER

SNACKS

FRIDAY

BREAKFAST

LUNCH

DINNER

SNACKS

SATURDAY

BREAKFAST

LUNCH

DINNER

SNACKS

SUNDAY

SHOPPING LIST

# DAY 57

DATE
| M | T | W | T | F | S | S |
|---|---|---|---|---|---|---|

Take care of your body. It's the only place you have to live.

 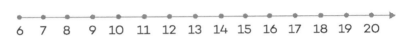

6  7  8  9  10  11  12  13  14  15  16  17  18  19  20

SLEEP    SLEEP QUALITY

ACTIVITY

BREAKFAST

SNACKS

LUNCH

TODAY I'M PROUD
OF MYSELF BECAUSE

DINNER

SOMETHING TO MAKE
TOMORROW BETTER?

I FEEL TODAY

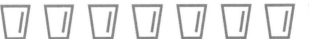

# DAY 58

If you're tired of starting over; stop giving up!

 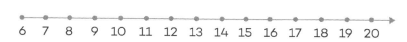

6   7   8   9   10   11   12   13   14   15   16   17   18   19   20

| SLEEP | SLEEP QUALITY  | ACTIVITY  |

BREAKFAST

SNACKS

LUNCH

TODAY I'M PROUD
OF MYSELF BECAUSE

DINNER

SOMETHING TO MAKE
TOMORROW BETTER?

I FEEL TODAY

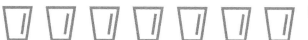

# DAY 59

On the other side of your workout is the body and health you want!

6  7  8  9  10  11  12  13  14  15  16  17  18  19  20

SLEEP    SLEEP QUALITY

ACTIVITY

BREAKFAST

SNACKS

LUNCH

TODAY I'M PROUD
OF MYSELF BECAUSE

DINNER

SOMETHING TO MAKE
TOMORROW BETTER?

I FEEL TODAY

# DAY 60

DATE
| M | T | W | T | F | S | S |
|---|---|---|---|---|---|---|
|   |   |   |   |   |   |   |

The question isn't can you, it's will you!

 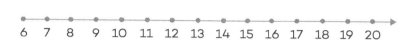

6   7   8   9   10   11   12   13   14   15   16   17   18   19   20

SLEEP        SLEEP QUALITY

ACTIVITY

BREAKFAST

SNACKS

LUNCH

TODAY I'M PROUD
OF MYSELF BECAUSE

DINNER

SOMETHING TO MAKE
TOMORROW BETTER?

I FEEL TODAY

       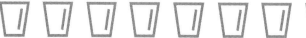

# DAY 61

Workouts are like life. The harder it is, the STRONGER YOU BECOME!

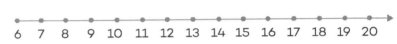

6  7  8  9  10  11  12  13  14  15  16  17  18  19  20

SLEEP    SLEEP QUALITY

ACTIVITY

BREAKFAST

SNACKS

LUNCH

TODAY I'M PROUD
OF MYSELF BECAUSE

DINNER

SOMETHING TO MAKE
TOMORROW BETTER?

I FEEL TODAY

# DAY 62

Don't wait until you've reached your goal to be proud of yourself.
Be proud of every step you take toward reaching that goal.

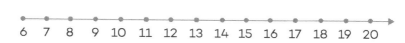

6 7 8 9 10 11 12 13 14 15 16 17 18 19 20

| SLEEP | SLEEP QUALITY  | ACTIVITY  |
|---|---|---|

**BREAKFAST**

**SNACKS**

**LUNCH**

**TODAY I'M PROUD OF MYSELF BECAUSE**

**DINNER**

**SOMETHING TO MAKE TOMORROW BETTER?**

I FEEL TODAY

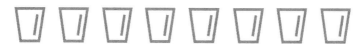

# DAY 63

DATE

| M | T | W | T | F | S | S |
|---|---|---|---|---|---|---|

If no one thinks you can, then you have to!

 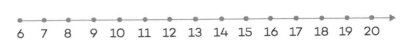

6 7 8 9 10 11 12 13 14 15 16 17 18 19 20

SLEEP          SLEEP QUALITY

ACTIVITY

BREAKFAST

SNACKS

LUNCH

TODAY I'M PROUD
OF MYSELF BECAUSE

DINNER

SOMETHING TO MAKE
TOMORROW BETTER?

I FEEL TODAY

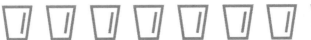

# WEEK 10 MEAL IDEAS

BREAKFAST

LUNCH

DINNER

SNACKS

**MONDAY**

BREAKFAST

LUNCH

DINNER

SNACKS

**TUESDAY**

BREAKFAST

LUNCH

DINNER

SNACKS

**WEDNESDAY**

BREAKFAST

LUNCH

DINNER

SNACKS

**THURSDAY**

BREAKFAST

LUNCH

DINNER

SNACKS

**FRIDAY**

BREAKFAST

LUNCH

DINNER

SNACKS

**SATURDAY**

BREAKFAST

LUNCH

DINNER

SNACKS

**SUNDAY**

SHOPPING LIST

# DAY 64

To enjoy the glow of good health, you must exercise.

 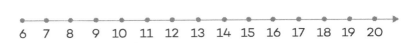

6  7  8  9  10  11  12  13  14  15  16  17  18  19  20

SLEEP        SLEEP QUALITY

ACTIVITY

BREAKFAST

SNACKS

LUNCH

TODAY I'M PROUD
OF MYSELF BECAUSE

DINNER

SOMETHING TO MAKE
TOMORROW BETTER?

I FEEL TODAY

     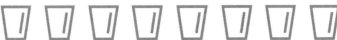

# DAY 65

DATE

| M | T | W | T | F | S | S |
|---|---|---|---|---|---|---|

If you still look good at the end of your work out-you didn't work hard enough!

 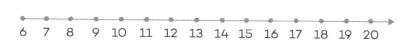

6  7  8  9  10  11  12  13  14  15  16  17  18  19  20

SLEEP        SLEEP QUALITY

ACTIVITY

BREAKFAST

SNACKS

LUNCH

TODAY I'M PROUD
OF MYSELF BECAUSE

DINNER

SOMETHING TO MAKE
TOMORROW BETTER?

I FEEL TODAY

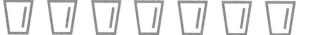

# DAY 66

You have to believe in yourself when no one else does
— that makes you a winner right there.

 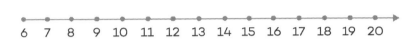

6  7  8  9  10  11  12  13  14  15  16  17  18  19  20

| SLEEP | SLEEP QUALITY  | ACTIVITY  |

| BREAKFAST | SNACKS |

| LUNCH | TODAY I'M PROUD OF MYSELF BECAUSE |

| DINNER | SOMETHING TO MAKE TOMORROW BETTER? |

I FEEL TODAY

# DAY 67

DATE

| M | T | W | T | F | S | S |

The hardest step to fitness is the first. Take it now!

 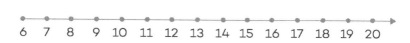

6  7  8  9  10  11  12  13  14  15  16  17  18  19  20

SLEEP    SLEEP QUALITY

ACTIVITY

BREAKFAST

SNACKS

LUNCH

TODAY I'M PROUD OF MYSELF BECAUSE

DINNER

SOMETHING TO MAKE TOMORROW BETTER?

I FEEL TODAY

       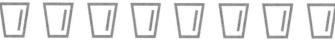

# DAY 68

DATE
| M | T | W | T | F | S | S |

Make time for it. Just get it done.
Nobody ever got strong or got in shape by thinking about it. They did it.

 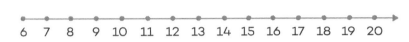

6  7  8  9  10  11  12  13  14  15  16  17  18  19  20

SLEEP       SLEEP QUALITY

ACTIVITY

BREAKFAST

SNACKS

LUNCH

TODAY I'M PROUD
OF MYSELF BECAUSE

DINNER

SOMETHING TO MAKE
TOMORROW BETTER?

I FEEL TODAY

     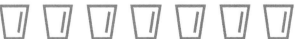

# DAY 69

Even if you are on the right track, you'll get run over if you just sit there.

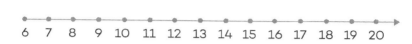

6  7  8  9  10  11  12  13  14  15  16  17  18  19  20

SLEEP        SLEEP QUALITY

ACTIVITY

BREAKFAST

SNACKS

LUNCH

TODAY I'M PROUD
OF MYSELF BECAUSE

DINNER

SOMETHING TO MAKE
TOMORROW BETTER?

I FEEL TODAY

# DAY 70

When you feel like quitting, think about why you started.

 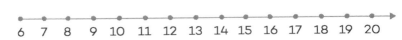

6  7  8  9  10  11  12  13  14  15  16  17  18  19  20

SLEEP    SLEEP QUALITY     ACTIVITY

BREAKFAST    SNACKS

LUNCH    TODAY I'M PROUD OF MYSELF BECAUSE

DINNER    SOMETHING TO MAKE TOMORROW BETTER?

I FEEL TODAY

# WEEK 11 MEAL IDEAS

## MONDAY
BREAKFAST

LUNCH

DINNER

SNACKS

## TUESDAY
BREAKFAST

LUNCH

DINNER

SNACKS

## WEDNESDAY
BREAKFAST

LUNCH

DINNER

SNACKS

## THURSDAY
BREAKFAST

LUNCH

DINNER

SNACKS

## FRIDAY
BREAKFAST

LUNCH

DINNER

SNACKS

## SATURDAY
BREAKFAST

LUNCH

DINNER

SNACKS

## SUNDAY
BREAKFAST

LUNCH

DINNER

SNACKS

## SHOPPING LIST

# DAY 71

Champions keep playing until they get it right.

 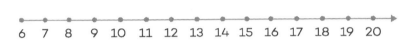

6  7  8  9  10  11  12  13  14  15  16  17  18  19  20

SLEEP    SLEEP QUALITY

ACTIVITY

BREAKFAST

SNACKS

LUNCH

TODAY I'M PROUD
OF MYSELF BECAUSE

DINNER

SOMETHING TO MAKE
TOMORROW BETTER?

I FEEL TODAY

# DAY 72

The hardest lift of all is lifting your butt off the couch.

 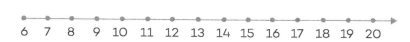

6  7  8  9  10  11  12  13  14  15  16  17  18  19  20

SLEEP        SLEEP QUALITY

ACTIVITY

BREAKFAST

SNACKS

LUNCH

TODAY I'M PROUD
OF MYSELF BECAUSE

DINNER

SOMETHING TO MAKE
TOMORROW BETTER?

I FEEL TODAY

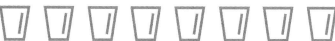

# DAY 73

DATE
| M | T | W | T | F | S | S |
|---|---|---|---|---|---|---|

Walking: the most ancient exercise and still the best modern exercise.

 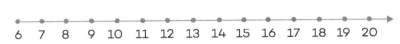

6  7  8  9  10  11  12  13  14  15  16  17  18  19  20

SLEEP    SLEEP QUALITY

ACTIVITY

BREAKFAST

SNACKS

LUNCH

TODAY I'M PROUD
OF MYSELF BECAUSE

DINNER

SOMETHING TO MAKE
TOMORROW BETTER?

I FEEL TODAY

     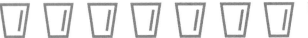

# DAY 74

DATE

| M | T | W | T | F | S | S |

Junk food you've craved for an hour, or the body you've craved for a lifetime? Your decision.

 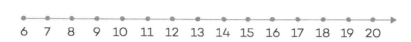

6  7  8  9  10  11  12  13  14  15  16  17  18  19  20

SLEEP          SLEEP QUALITY

ACTIVITY

BREAKFAST

SNACKS

LUNCH

TODAY I'M PROUD OF MYSELF BECAUSE

DINNER

SOMETHING TO MAKE TOMORROW BETTER?

I FEEL TODAY

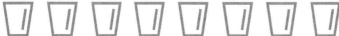

# DAY 75

If it doesn't challenge you, it doesn't change you.

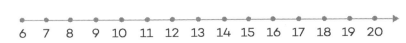

6  7  8  9  10  11  12  13  14  15  16  17  18  19  20

SLEEP    SLEEP QUALITY

ACTIVITY

BREAKFAST

SNACKS

LUNCH

TODAY I'M PROUD
OF MYSELF BECAUSE

DINNER

SOMETHING TO MAKE
TOMORROW BETTER?

I FEEL TODAY

# DAY 76

DATE

| M | T | W | T | F | S | S |
|---|---|---|---|---|---|---|

Losing weight is a mind game. Change your mind. Change your body.

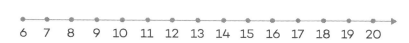

6  7  8  9  10  11  12  13  14  15  16  17  18  19  20

SLEEP          SLEEP QUALITY

ACTIVITY

BREAKFAST

SNACKS

LUNCH

TODAY I'M PROUD
OF MYSELF BECAUSE

DINNER

SOMETHING TO MAKE
TOMORROW BETTER?

I FEEL TODAY

# DAY 77

Nobody can do it for you, you have to do it yourself.

  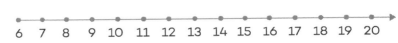

6  7  8  9  10  11  12  13  14  15  16  17  18  19  20

SLEEP      SLEEP QUALITY            ACTIVITY

BREAKFAST                          SNACKS

LUNCH                              TODAY I'M PROUD
                                   OF MYSELF BECAUSE

DINNER                             SOMETHING TO MAKE
                                   TOMORROW BETTER?

I FEEL TODAY

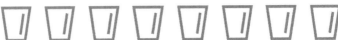

# WEEK 12 MEAL IDEAS

| MONDAY | |
|---|---|
| BREAKFAST | |
| LUNCH | |
| DINNER | |
| SNACKS | |

| TUESDAY | |
|---|---|
| BREAKFAST | |
| LUNCH | |
| DINNER | |
| SNACKS | |

| WEDNESDAY | |
|---|---|
| BREAKFAST | |
| LUNCH | |
| DINNER | |
| SNACKS | |

| THURSDAY | |
|---|---|
| BREAKFAST | |
| LUNCH | |
| DINNER | |
| SNACKS | |

| FRIDAY | |
|---|---|
| BREAKFAST | |
| LUNCH | |
| DINNER | |
| SNACKS | |

| SATURDAY | |
|---|---|
| BREAKFAST | |
| LUNCH | |
| DINNER | |
| SNACKS | |

| SUNDAY | |
|---|---|
| BREAKFAST | |
| LUNCH | |
| DINNER | |
| SNACKS | |

SHOPPING LIST

# DAY 78

Pain is temporary, quitting lasts forever.

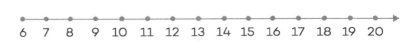

6  7  8  9  10  11  12  13  14  15  16  17  18  19  20

SLEEP        SLEEP QUALITY

ACTIVITY

BREAKFAST

SNACKS

LUNCH

TODAY I'M PROUD
OF MYSELF BECAUSE

DINNER

SOMETHING TO MAKE
TOMORROW BETTER?

I FEEL TODAY

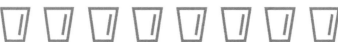

# DAY 79

DATE

| M | T | W | T | F | S | S |
|---|---|---|---|---|---|---|

A one hour workout is 4% of your day. No excuses!

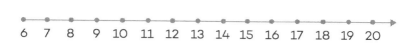

6   7   8   9   10   11   12   13   14   15   16   17   18   19   20

SLEEP          SLEEP QUALITY             ACTIVITY

BREAKFAST                                      SNACKS

LUNCH                                          TODAY I'M PROUD
                                               OF MYSELF BECAUSE

DINNER                                         SOMETHING TO MAKE
                                               TOMORROW BETTER?

I FEEL TODAY

# DAY 80

DATE

| M | T | W | T | F | S | S |
|---|---|---|---|---|---|---|
|   |   |   |   |   |   |   |

Good things come to those who work.

 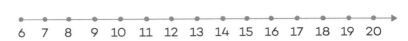

6  7  8  9  10  11  12  13  14  15  16  17  18  19  20

SLEEP    SLEEP QUALITY

ACTIVITY

BREAKFAST

SNACKS

LUNCH

TODAY I'M PROUD
OF MYSELF BECAUSE

DINNER

SOMETHING TO MAKE
TOMORROW BETTER?

I FEEL TODAY

# DAY 81

DATE

| M | T | W | T | F | S | S |
|---|---|---|---|---|---|---|

Slow progress is better than no progress.

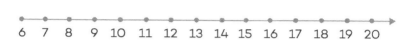

6  7  8  9  10  11  12  13  14  15  16  17  18  19  20

SLEEP      SLEEP QUALITY

ACTIVITY

BREAKFAST

SNACKS

LUNCH

TODAY I'M PROUD
OF MYSELF BECAUSE

DINNER

SOMETHING TO MAKE
TOMORROW BETTER?

I FEEL TODAY

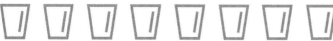

# DAY 82

One of the great moments in life is realizing that two weeks ago
your body couldn't do what it just did.

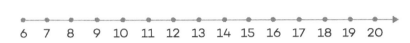

6  7  8  9  10  11  12  13  14  15  16  17  18  19  20

| SLEEP          SLEEP QUALITY  | ACTIVITY  |
|---|---|
| BREAKFAST | SNACKS |
| LUNCH | TODAY I'M PROUD OF MYSELF BECAUSE |
| DINNER | SOMETHING TO MAKE TOMORROW BETTER? |

I FEEL TODAY

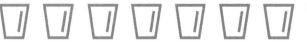

# DAY 83

Your desire to change must be greater than your desire to stay the same.

 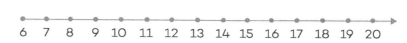

6  7  8  9  10  11  12  13  14  15  16  17  18  19  20

| SLEEP | SLEEP QUALITY  | ACTIVITY  |
|---|---|---|

BREAKFAST

SNACKS

LUNCH

TODAY I'M PROUD
OF MYSELF BECAUSE

DINNER

SOMETHING TO MAKE
TOMORROW BETTER?

I FEEL TODAY

       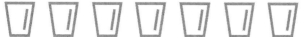

# DAY 84

DATE

| M | T | W | T | F | S | S |
|---|---|---|---|---|---|---|

If you're tired of starting over then stop giving up.

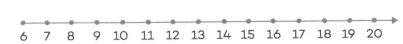

6  7  8  9  10  11  12  13  14  15  16  17  18  19  20

SLEEP     SLEEP QUALITY

ACTIVITY

BREAKFAST

SNACKS

LUNCH

TODAY I'M PROUD
OF MYSELF BECAUSE

DINNER

SOMETHING TO MAKE
TOMORROW BETTER?

I FEEL TODAY

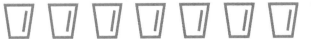

# WEEK 13 MEAL IDEAS

| | MONDAY |
|---|---|
| BREAKFAST | |
| LUNCH | |
| DINNER | |
| SNACKS | |

| | TUESDAY |
|---|---|
| BREAKFAST | |
| LUNCH | |
| DINNER | |
| SNACKS | |

| | WEDNESDAY |
|---|---|
| BREAKFAST | |
| LUNCH | |
| DINNER | |
| SNACKS | |

| | THURSDAY |
|---|---|
| BREAKFAST | |
| LUNCH | |
| DINNER | |
| SNACKS | |

| | FRIDAY |
|---|---|
| BREAKFAST | |
| LUNCH | |
| DINNER | |
| SNACKS | |

| | SATURDAY |
|---|---|
| BREAKFAST | |
| LUNCH | |
| DINNER | |
| SNACKS | |

| | SUNDAY |
|---|---|
| BREAKFAST | |
| LUNCH | |
| DINNER | |
| SNACKS | |

SHOPPING LIST

# DAY 85

To give anything less than your best is to sacrifice the gift.

 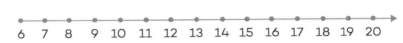

6  7  8  9  10  11  12  13  14  15  16  17  18  19  20

SLEEP    SLEEP QUALITY

ACTIVITY

BREAKFAST

SNACKS

LUNCH

TODAY I'M PROUD
OF MYSELF BECAUSE

DINNER

SOMETHING TO MAKE
TOMORROW BETTER?

I FEEL TODAY

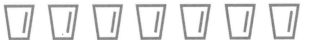

# DAY 86

DATE

| M | T | W | T | F | S | S |
|---|---|---|---|---|---|---|
|   |   |   |   |   |   |   |

Losing weight is hard. Being overweight is hard. Choose your hard.

6  7  8  9  10  11  12  13  14  15  16  17  18  19  20

| SLEEP    SLEEP QUALITY  | ACTIVITY  |
|---|---|

| BREAKFAST | SNACKS |
|---|---|

| LUNCH | TODAY I'M PROUD OF MYSELF BECAUSE |
|---|---|

| DINNER | SOMETHING TO MAKE TOMORROW BETTER? |
|---|---|

I FEEL TODAY

# DAY 87

Exercise to be fit, not skinny. Eat to nourish your body and always ignore the haters. You are worth more than you realise.

 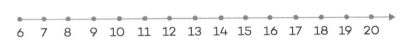

6  7  8  9  10  11  12  13  14  15  16  17  18  19  20

| SLEEP | SLEEP QUALITY  | ACTIVITY  |
|---|---|---|

BREAKFAST

SNACKS

LUNCH

TODAY I'M PROUD OF MYSELF BECAUSE

DINNER

SOMETHING TO MAKE TOMORROW BETTER?

I FEEL TODAY

# DAY 88

You only fail when you stop trying.

6  7  8  9  10  11  12  13  14  15  16  17  18  19  20

SLEEP     SLEEP QUALITY

ACTIVITY

BREAKFAST

SNACKS

LUNCH

TODAY I'M PROUD
OF MYSELF BECAUSE

DINNER

SOMETHING TO MAKE
TOMORROW BETTER?

I FEEL TODAY

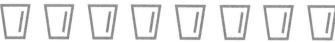

# DAY 89

DATE

| M | T | W | T | F | S | S |
|---|---|---|---|---|---|---|

Eat for the body you want. Not for the body you have.

 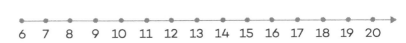

6 7 8 9 10 11 12 13 14 15 16 17 18 19 20

SLEEP  SLEEP QUALITY

ACTIVITY

BREAKFAST

SNACKS

LUNCH

TODAY I'M PROUD
OF MYSELF BECAUSE

DINNER

SOMETHING TO MAKE
TOMORROW BETTER?

I FEEL TODAY

       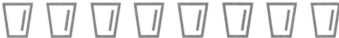

# DAY 90

DATE _____

| M | T | W | T | F | S | S |

You get what you work for, not what you wish for.

 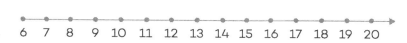

6  7  8  9  10  11  12  13  14  15  16  17  18  19  20

SLEEP          SLEEP QUALITY

ACTIVITY

BREAKFAST

SNACKS

LUNCH

TODAY I'M PROUD
OF MYSELF BECAUSE

DINNER

SOMETHING TO MAKE
TOMORROW BETTER?

I FEEL TODAY

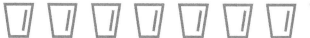

# Congratulations!
# YOU DID IT!

> IT ALWAYS SEEMS
> # IMPOSSIBLE
> UNTIL IT'S DONE

Made in the USA
Middletown, DE
13 February 2022

61052834R00066